SURVIVING CANCER
AT BOTH ENDS

By
Bob Crew

Powerful poetry from the killing fields of cancer about the nature of mouth cancer and prostate cancer and how one survivor has survived these diseases for eleven years.

Paperback ISBN 978-1-80424-172-1
ePub ISBN 978-1-80424-173-8
PDF ISBN 978-1-80424-174-5

Published by MX Publishing
335 Princess Park Manor, Royal Drive,
London, N11 3GX
www.mxpublishing.com

Cover design by Brian Belanger

Neil Vickers, **Lecturer in Literature and Medicine at King's College, University of London**: '*Cancer at Both Ends has tremendous value. It is rare to find real poetry on these subjects. This is subtle and powerful verse. Really terrific. I admire the strength of character, the humour and the willingness to embrace the very uncomfortable truth that there is no reason why we should not get cancer. Wonderful poetry.*'

Michael Lee, 2003 Editor of *Poems in the* **Waiting** *Room*: '*Cancer at Both Ends is a remarkable collection – an impressive, stirring record. Medicine has been classically defined as the study of the progress of disease through the morbid anatomy. Bob Crew's work is a healthy response. It is exceptionally strong and moving with a life-giving touch of humour.*

Professor Michael Baum, Cancer Surgeon and former Professor of Surgery at Kings College Hospital, Royal Marsden Hospital and University College Hospital. *'Wonderful and deeply moving.'*

James Poole, BA Natural Sciences (Cambridge): *'It's kind of awesome that the Big C creates opportunities for such savage humour and irony. Bob Crew's humour is not just mischievous, it's contagious. He has also put his finger on a very interesting area of intellectual debate – Complexity Theory. The wonder is not why things go wrong, but that they do not. But why does it take only one molecule going awl, or wrong, to cause big bad cancer?'*

Preface

The following collection of thirty-four mouth and prostate cancer poems is written from my personal experience as a cancer sufferer and survivor and also from several conversations I have had with maxillofacial cancer surgeons Lawrence Newman and Nicholas Kalavrezos, radiography professor Michelle Saunders, and dental surgeon Mark Barrett - all part of the same maxillofacial team at University College Hospital in Central London where I began to receive horrendous cancer treatments in 2003 – and also with Amir Kaisary, consultant urologist at the Royal Free Hospital at Hampstead in North London on the subject of prostate cancer, for which I was under surveillance and eventually had key surgery, also in 2003. This was almost immediately after Lawrence Newman and his team operated on my neck for mouth cancer. It is no exaggeration to say that I have been in a bloody war with cancer since 2003, having come out of remission in 2005 when peace was finally declared!

But war broke out once again in 2020 – 19 years later – when cancer returned to me at the other bottom-end of my body between my legs (ha-ha) this time in the form of an incurable, red alert Grade-A-Advanced Prostate Cancer, that is slowly and gradually killing me off, as I speak. And once again I am back in the excellent care of University College Hospital London, being monitored and treated by Professor Michelle Roberts, Dr Anita Mitra and *Clinical Nurse Extraordinaire*, Karen Wilkinson; another brilliant team, to be sure, taking over from the Head and Neck people previously, the leader of whom, the aforementioned Lawrence Newman, prophetically observed back in 2003 that cancer does sometimes (mischievously!) return in a different guise later on, to have two bites at the cherry, or a walnut (gland) in my case.

Rotten luck and tough luck indeed!

Nineteen years and more is a lot of rotten and tough luck to endure, but it has had its golden moments, and I am still actively working, soldiering on globetrotting, for all that, and not letting the lethal and scary dangers of this pesky disease get me down (why would I not?), as I increasingly think about my approaching death and the meaning of life with a continuing smile on my face (why would I not?),

Having, for these reasons, discovered that there are un-ignorable things happening in the killing fields of cancer that can be addressed to good effect in poetry - in the same way that war poets have, in their time, written about their battlefield experiences in the military theatres of war – I have written this collection of poems.

A goodly number of these un-ignorable things are addressed in these pages in blank verse, free verse, sprung verse and rhyming verse, all different styles to suit different purposes and moods. When I received my two English Literature degrees – BA (Hons), MA – from the university of London, I of course never imagined that all the lovely poetry I enjoyed reading (and occasionally writing) would inspire me to write about such a grim and ugly gloom and doom disease as cancer! But we must all rise above life's gloom and doom and diseases and, remember that, as Oscar Wilde once said, when we find ourselves lying in the cutter, for whatever reason, we can always look at the stars (as I never fail to do in so many different ways),

I was invited to read the first poem in this collection – 'Poetry of the Poisoned Mouth' – to members of parliament and the medical and dental professions at the House of Commons in aid of a Mouth Cancer Awareness Week.

Whilst none of the poetry in this collection is for the faint-hearted, cancer is not for the faint-hearted either, and there is no reason why we should not get to grips with it in poetry as well as in prose. Hideous as it is, deeply and painfully personal experience of suffering a cancer can be transformed with poetry and to very good effect (albeit not beatified, of course not).

Whilst cancer does atrociously victimise us, for sure, we don't have to settle for the lowly mindset of a victim; on the contrary we can, if we prefer, triumphantly rise above it with whatever it takes to rise above it, not just with poetry, but with whatever else it is in our higher and better nature to inspire us to do so.

Trust me, I know what I'm talking about.

Bob Crew
Hampstead Garden Suburb,
North London
December 2022,

Contents

Poetry of the Poisoned Mouth

A crab crawled out
from under my tongue
to play a tune on a mouth organ,
a colourless tune, liquid white
as a ghost that haunted me
with a message from hell
encoded in tissues of skin
with a horror story to tell,
swelling tissues,
swiftly turning
like pages written
in some kind of cipher
and hard at the core.

I went to see a code breaker
who introduced me to an expert
knife-man who obligingly slit my throat
from ear to Adam's Apple, for this was
no zodiacal crab. This was the other sort.
A biting crab, aggressive, vicious and nasty.

*This poem was read by Bob Crew to MPs and cancer and
dental surgeons at the House of Commonsin
in November 2007at the launch of Mouth Cancer Awareness
Week.*

Wiping the 2003 Smile from Your Face

One death every five hours
is enough to wipe the smile
from your face as 6,000 new victims
go down with oral cancer every year,
twice as many men as women,
and children too, a five-year old
in Birmingham, just recently.

People say they are lost for words
when their friends and colleagues
go down with it and maybe lose
their voices and also their lives
in due course. I lost my voice
for a while, but not for long,
and not my life either.

Oncology

The scientific study of tumours is called oncology,
which is a subject that makes no apology
for losing a battle that it cannot hope to win,
as it takes its defeat so valiantly on the chin.

What need is there of apology when the medics have fought
a good fight and made sure to do all they've been taught?

There is no need,
so God speed!

Tumours are a hideous mass of abnormal tissues
growing where they ought not to be growing
in so many different parts of our bodies.

Atrocious are the personal insults that a tumour issues,
as it mocks, ridicules and humiliates its victims, throwing
everything it has at them in the way of deadly maladies.

Most cancer patients have never heard this oncology word
before. To them this mystifying word is quite absurd!

Cancer they sort of understand,
death and disease they understand,
suffering they understand.

But oncology
is a perplexing ology
about which they
know not what to say.

A Visit to the Maxillofacial Department

Sitting in the maxillofacial reception
of London's University College Hospital
I feel that my face may turn into a mess
of distorted and disfigured shock-horror
flesh and bone that could eventually
give me and passers-by a dreadful fright
out of the dark night of my diseased head
every time I look into a startled mirror
and crack it, or into the eyes of others
and smack them with an ugly mug
to stop a clock!

I feel the tears of blood
welling up in my eyes
as I sit in this reception
surrounded by such faces
far worse than mine,
as they beckon
my possible future
and my fears.

Frozen tears and ice-cold
blood, no fuss and no mess
in the hot red for danger
passion of my emotions.

I feel the skeletal mask
of the Grim Reaper
pushed in my face
by the rude hand of death
to make a perfect fit -
let's hope I scare him
more than he scares me! –

as it happens he does not,
truth to tell, scare me at all.
Gutsy to the last, that's me.
I'll take my chances with death
any day, any time, you'll see.

On the other hand,
perhaps this is easy to say,
until the appointed day.

I fail to understand what I –
what any maxillofacial patient –
has done to deserve this savage
cancer, as we all compete with
The Grim Reaper for the ugliest
mug in town!

As yet, my mug is not ugly
at all – my neck is scarred
that's all! – but as we know
from the statistics only 5%
of mouth cancer patients
survive, as I seem to be
doing, thus far.

I am one of those who can look
on the bright side, whilst also
looking over my shoulder
at the dark side
of the moon.

But should the ghastly time come
for me to join the freak show
with a heavy heart
and a twisted face,

I'm out of here fast!

Please don't ask me to hang around
in the interests of friends and family
or modern medicine with cancer's final insult
written all over my face without apparent reason.

Please don't heap this humiliation on me of all people!

As I see it, this is too much to ask, needlessly breaking
your hearts and becoming a burden to all, including myself!

Nothing personal, but I'll be on my way,
if it's all the same to you, as I sincerely hope
that it will be, if you read this poem carefully.
As for my nearest and dearest, they will know
that it's not personal at all.

Knowing and loving me –
ha, ha! - they will understand
that I love them far too much
to put them through any more
of this crap. They will comprehend
that I am too stylish and too clever
for such a disease as oral cancer
which will not have the last laugh
on me – you'll see.

If things get worse,
I'll cheat the ugly beast
by bravely and honourably
giving myself to euthanasia

instead of hanging around
to become a sight for sore eyes
and a final stab in the heart
to loved ones, a final fist
in my face, and for whose benefit,
I should really like to know?

Not mine, not yours, not anybody's
that we can think of. So let me go
to my death with a clear conscience
and a brave and proud heart.

What's wrong with that?

Who needs all this humiliation
and pain and ugliness at the end
of an otherwise good and handsome life?

If handsome is what handsome does,
what did I or anybody else do?
Don't all answer at once!

Life is largely a joke
that dare not speak
its name, and we know
this, in our hearts,
to be true as we turn
an eternally blind eye
to the misery, the inequality
and inanity, as we hope for
the best!

On the other hand,
it is also no joke at all,
and this defies belief, as a rule.

But how are we to account
metaphysically for all
the cruel diseases
that give us a kick
up the tireless rump
on our way out?

What is the nature of existence
and the truth of knowledge
supposed to be about?

What on earth has it to do with
cancer and other fatal diseases?

As I say, don't all answer at once!

Cheerfully or Otherwise

Cheerfully or otherwise
we must all expect to die
from one thing or another,
so who cares if it's cancer?

Death comes as no surprise,
it's an inescapable fact of life, so why
fret? But excruciating torture by a vicious cancer,
or some other nasty disease, is certainly extra bother!

Even so, if that's how the cookie crumbles, bring it on, say I,
as I do my feeble best to see if I cannot hold my head high!

Bewildered

I am told that cancer of the mouth
or throat is caused by having a gene
that makes you vulnerable to the
disease and then by smoking like
a chimney and boozing too much.

The smoking and boozing trigger the cancer
that is not possible without the necessary gene.

But I have never smoked
a single cigarette in my life.
Nor have I been a binge drinker.

Bewildering, isn't it?

Or is it?

Cunnilingus is also said to be a cause
and I've done plenty of that.

Oh yes, I've been a *cunnilinguist
extraordinaire*, tipping the velvet
this way and that, paying lip service
to women in this way, risking that fatal
virus from the cervix, of which we were
not aware in earlier years, and if that is
the cause, then I have no regrets.

It was all worth it!

Choose Your Parents Carefully!

When an inherited susceptibility
to the disease is triggered
by carcinogenic, dietary
or environmental factors
– carcinogenic meaning
chemicals, radiation or
viruses – then Big Bad Cancer
will have its wicked way with us,
unless, it seems, we give up smoking,
drinking alcohol, eating favourite foods,
sun bathing and sex, and what is
more we should take good care
to choose our parents carefully!

But neither my mother
nor father had cancer,
although their mothers did.

Secretive Fruit

The fig is indeed a secretive fruit,
dear Lawrence, as the Italians have
suggested, with its inward flowering
and its quivering fibres that are so
moist and womb-like and deliciously
fleshy and juicy with it, such a perfect
fit through a single orifice, and so
tempting to lick and to suck and then
to fuck en-route to cancer of the mouth
maybe – that last secret of all – if your
luck is out when your tongue is in.

Unignorable

It's best not to dwell
on two years of hell
and the unrelenting discomfort of yet another three
until, fingers crossed, you're finally mouth-cancer free.

Not two months of hell, *but two years*,
frozen solid in ice-cold tears,
as you hold your shrinking-stinking breath
and think far too much about death.

Now there's a thought
that will come to nought!

Yet you cannot ignore the unignorable.
You need to dwell on it, however deplorable.

So let every detail of the prolonged misery
be transformed into some harrowing poetry,
if indeed you are a poet
and know how to hack it
in those dark places where
there is nothing but despair.

Not all cancers are as vicious or anywhere near as devastating
as others, but they are all potentially deadly and withering,
and of course there are some other diseases that are almost
or just as bad. But, as for mouth cancer, it is by far the most
invasive, excruciating and deadly
and it was nearly the death of me.

When Larkin had oral cancer he chickened out
of letting his poetry have the last shout.

He died of the disease in 1985, but when it came to me,
in 2003, I met it head on with my poetry.

My word! The power of the pen.
Perhaps it is mightier than the sword.

But it's not possible to write one's self out of death
and cancer is it? Don't hold your breath.

Loose Ends and Nerve Ends

The flesh in my neck
                    is crawling with
stinging nettles
                that grow wild
like bracken
                down to my chest
and over the top
                of my back.
They are all over my
                    neck, chest, shoulders
and upper back
                like an invisible rash
in remembrance
                    of my cancer treatment
and the pain-killers
                    that can sort it
make me dizzy
                so I do not use them.

There are stick-on pain killing
                            patches that I could use
but they are tiresome
                        and have a habit of falling off
under my clothes
                so I don't use them either.

It seems that my shattered and tattered
                                nerve ends
are healing inside my flesh
                            after too much radiotherapy
and the surgeon's knife
                        and it feels as though
I have a heavy strap

                    round the back of my neck
pulling it down
                    with my chin
gesturing towards
                    my chest.
I try to remember
                    to hold my neck up straight
but this is also tiresome
                            and I often forget
in remembrance of my cancer
                                    in this never to be forgotten
sting and ring of time
                    that is now five years old.

Tiresome is the word.
                    These after effects get you down.
They tire and irritate
                    in the nerve-racking sting
and echoing ring of time.
                            But the story does not end there!
There are stabbing pains
                    in my jaws
and aches deeply embedded
                            in my ear drums!!
In fact the story
                    is a load of crap
that has fallen
                    into my lap
for whatever reason
                            crap falls on us
in this life.
            How to handle the crap
and survive it
                    is what the story
is all about.

Not what it means.
Don't look for meanings
in a story
of this kind.

Thou shalt not smoke
chew or drink alcohol
or tongue women?
Thou shalt suffer
and die
without asking why?
Thou shalt
drop dead
and consider yourself lucky
if you die in your bed?
Listen:
whatever this story is about -
morbid
anatomies and so on –
it aint going to
make much sense
because there are
too many loose ends
and nerve ends
and mouth cancer victims
dying
at the rate of one person
every five hours
in Britain alone.

A Visit to the Mould Room

A Visit to the Mould Room
to have your cheerful face
smothered in wet but warm
Plaster of Paris - that takes ten
minutes to capture an impression
of your features – is essential to protect
the front of your head from the blistering
radioactive rays that are going to blitz it
to hell and back in their vicious assault
on your mouth cancer that is pulling a face
at you! But don't be blue! You may beat it yet.

Women lose their makeup in the plaster
and bearded men are required to shave
their bristly hairs, while both need to cut
the hair on their heads short so that it does not
get in the way of the impression that is taken.

When the plaster has set,
it is lifted off in one piece,
leaving you to wash away
any remaining traces,
but not, alas, your cares.

It takes a couple of days more
for your mould to turn into
see-though fibreglass plastic
and, if it fits, then you are ready
to do battle, like a medieval Knight
from days of old, in his helmet!

Make no mistake about it.
It is one hell of a barbaric battle

that is about to commence…..

Holes have been left for your eyes,
nose and mouth, and a pimply rash
of bullet holes have been strategically
and neatly perforated on both sides
of your neck, into and under your jaw
on the right side and between your
left shoulder and breast.

These are carefully targeted holes
to which the radioactive rays will be
computer-directed when the battle
commences - a fight to the death,
win or lose! But don't be blue!
You may beat it yet.

By directing the radioactive rays
into these bull's eye holes,
your surrounding skin
and flesh is protected
from collateral damage
that would otherwise
leave you looking
and feeling like
a Chernobyl victim!

But nothing can protect you
from internal collateral damage
inside your sandpit-dry mouth
and throat after glands have been
cut way and saliva has gone missing.
Or from the damage to your teeth
long after the battle is over, when

stripped of their enamel by the mini
atomic explosions in your oral cavity
that have caused your teeth to decay,
splinter and crumble – explosions that
can rip flesh from your infected gums
right down to your jaw bone –
your formerly healthy fangs
are need of a dentist fast!

Throughout your intensive radiotherapy treatment,
you will wear your mould daily, like a scary mask,
five days a week and for at least six weeks or more,
depending on the progress you make, and before long
the smile will be wiped from your now frowning face,
which is not the end of the world, because the party's
not over until it's over!

And if, as your friends and loved ones hope
and pray, you win to fight another day,
you will not be able to eat for six months
on account of your tongue feeling as though
it has been slashed with razors, and your throat
feeling as though it has a lump of barbed wire
inserted in it to prevent swallowing, and your neck
feeling as though it has lumps of wood and/or cardboard
inserted in it, as you vomit daily for a record-breaking
sixteen days, right round the clock, with a sick bucket
at your bedside, while you are fed liquid nutrients
through a slender tube pegged into your stomach!

Which is why you will have massive night sweats,
which is why you will lose at least three stone in weight.

And it all began with an interesting visit to the Mould Room where medics skilfully plastered your face to take an impression of its features, but not of your suffering, stamina or brave heart, because it seems that they have no moulds or impressions for such things, each of which have to be your own work!

As we see, it is also your character that is being moulded here, but not in the Mould Room. So take heart, because if this cancer doesn't kill you, it will certainly strengthen you, that's for sure.

Enough is Enough

Most cancer of the mouth sufferers
are massively exhausted
under the sledge-hammer blow
of the disease and the treatment.

They can hardly keep their eyes open
to receive their radiotherapy
when they drag themselves
to hospital each day.

When they return home
they are crushed into sleep
for hours of night sweats
and day sweats.

Some are so pulverised
by exhaustion -
physical, mental
and emotional -
and driven so deep
into depression
on account of it,
that they soon feel
that they cannot go on,
that enough is enough.

Eaten Alive

It's as if you are being eaten alive
by your own mouth, as if your teeth
have turned against you and are making a meal
of the inside of your face instead of the usual foods!

As you live this nightmare, your mouth does a savage u-turn
and eats you up from inside itself, devouring its own tongue
as well as the lining of your oral cavity, plunging its fangs
deep down into what feels like a petrified and disappearing
throat!

It's a ravenous mouth that has suddenly turned against itself,
just as the bad cancer cells in your body have turned against
the good cells, and your life has turned against you, as you try
to decide where you stand in all this, in relation to yourself,
watching your self-image image disappear
down the plug hole of your hungry mouth…..

It's as if your mouth may eat your head off
before it's through!

As your mouth eats itself and you away,
it is also as if you are in retreat, falling backwards
down the well of your throat, where you may
finish up being eaten alive!

The tender lining of your throat
is closer to you than your skin.
It's like a silky under-skin
with a sensitive outer touch
that tears easily like the flesh
of a soft peach

soaked in juice
of acid pain.

Nothing poisons the mouth like cancer,
as it spreads like salt in the wound,
not only of your oral cavity,
but also of your heart and soul.
So be brave of heart
and strong of mind
and let your soul
look after itself.

Up Against It

You may have noticed that
I am not circling round cancer
lightly – like a pretty butterfly
hovering from flower to flower,
or a shadow gently touching a person
on the shoulder – on the contrary I am
confronting the beast head on and looking
at it close-up, as it is already in my face
and at my throat, seven days a week!

I am engaged, not in shadow boxing,
but the real thing, as I grapple with
the disease and the suffering it inflicts,
writing my poetry about it so that it can
become knowable and understandable,
not least in terms of the humanity that
is still possible in the ugly face of the
otherwise impossible inhumanity of it all!

When you have had your head stuck
in a sick bucket at your bedside
for sixteen long days, right round
the clock, and been almost washed
away by massive sink-or-swim night sweats,
you realise that you are up against cancer,
not circling round it, and when you write
your poetry, you fire real bullets, not blanks,
as you take careful aim. As time runs out,
you leave nothing out, as you pay attention
to detail in your desperate attempts to nail
cancer, which sure as hell is nailing you.

This is too much like hard work to be
cathartic, but it is informative
and revealing, and it is not
impossible that such
unpalatable truths told
in poetry may actually
be good for readers.

Too many poets have ignored cancer
for too long, whilst others have not
got up to their elbows, deep into it,
or under its skin. They have not
discovered its ugly fascination!

Becoming Cancer

You suddenly feel as though you are
a symptom of cancer rather than
an actual person.

You feel like a mere sign of the existence
of an alien condition that has nothing
to do with the real you.

You no longer feel like an actual
person, but a strange indication
of a person, a diseased person.

You feel like
an injured soul.
Proper poorly
and not yourself!

You feel,
not only
that you
have the
symptom,
but that
you *are*
the symptom,
that cancer becomes you,
as you become cancer!

You feel depersonalised
and even after it has
apparently gone away,
when you are in remission,
you feel that you are not

out of gaol yet.

You feel as though
there is an ominous
lodger in the house
of your body –
an impostor –
who will be
the death
of you
if he
is not
evicted.

But how to evict him?

Heroic Memories

To remember who you are
when vile cancer inflicts its
atrocious pain and ugliness
upon you is one hell of a thing
to remember!

But if you can remember that
you are not the ugly spectacle
that cancer has made of you,
if you can resist becoming
your pain and your ugliness,
then you will also remember that
you are that beautiful or handsome
pain-free person that you always
were and still are in your heart
and soul that is beyond the
contamination of cancer.

You will retain
your massive dignity
amidst the deeply
dishonest and unjust
indignity doled out
by cancer.

But these are seriously heroic memories indeed
that will not come easily in your time of need.

You will have to work at them,
just as your doctors and surgeons
are working at your survival.

Nothing is for nothing

or achieved without effort.

Scanned to Death

These scans that search through
every component part of your body,
turning it inside out and revealing
it nakedly in magnificent monochrome,
dissecting it image by image, and probing
like an army of tireless glow worms
in the all-pervading dark of night,
lighting up the hidden places
of your mysterious inner sanctum
between and inside your ears,
under and over your tongue,
down your throat and up your bum,
into the deepest recesses of your heart,
inside your underclothes, in and out
of your pancreas, liver and womb,
up your nose, through your breasts
and your chest, into your lungs,
under your arms and between
your legs and your toes,
they know no bounds,
these unstoppable scans.

They may even stop you from dying,
from whatever it is that you're dying,
but if not, it won't be for the want of trying.

And when you have been scanned to death -
after taking but not scanning your last breath -
when you are long gone,

and no longer belong,
these scans will have you on file
and maybe for quite a while,
unless you take their images
with you, as visual spillages
of your remains
out of your veins
and into the flames
or the grave.

Camouflage

For fear of evaporation,
people generally deny
their feelings, not least
doctors and surgeons who,
with their evasive language,
are at risk of feeling and saying
too little because they have
too much to feel and to fear,
as they struggle to save their
patients' lives, watching some
go over the top, never to return,
and others lingering painfully
in their embattled trenches
that are camouflaged as
sick beds, just as feelings
are also camouflaged as
hope, never say die and
no surrender when there
really is not a hope in hell
(otherwise patients who are
not free to go would be free
to go)!

Then there are those visitors
who do not deny their feelings
at all, but cry all over patients
instead, because they say they
cannot help it, as if their crying
is supposed to be good for patients
and is going to save them or make
them feel better (if only!). Not for these
visitors any camouflage, and no doubt

their crying makes patients feel worse,
because they have enough upset and anxiety
of their own to worry about and do not need
to be distracted and disturbed therefore
by crumpled sheets of uncomfortable
tears, unless they are past caring,
which is all too the good.
But maybe the crying makes
the tearful visitors feel better.

As for nurses, rushing from bed to bed,
it is hardly surprising if, to most of them,
their patients are not much more than numbers
and a lot of hard work they could do without
as each tiresome bed bug – full of illness and
infection from whom the nurses get no relief
- waits in line to be called by that old Grim Reaper,
old as time, with all the time in the world, himself
camouflaged by a shock-horror costume that may
or may not be genuine, as he plays to his audience.

These nurses have feelings
to camouflage also, as they
attend to patients with camouflaged
smiles they do not mean, that are
stuck over their uncomplaining
mouths like sticky plaster, as they
swallow their complaints as they
are required to do, swallowing them
with their dignity in order not to be rude
before they die, in order not to let themselves
down or be discourteous to their visitors,
in order to practise one last time the gentle art
of camouflage, as their emotions are tightly
folded away like bed sheets with neat and tidy

envelope corners, making them presentable
for death, as they try to scrub up well!

There are also visitors who irritate
by telling patients how well they
look, when they look like sickly
scarecrows, and there are other
visitors who say that things are
going to be alright when they
are obviously going badly,
or when nobody has any
idea if such optimism
is in any way justified.

To add insult to injury,
there are those who never
much liked or cared about
patients but nevertheless
regularly ask them - when
they see them on the street
if they should become out
patients – how they are,
wishing them well and also
asking after them when
formerly they could not have
cared less. Maybe they have
a bad conscience, or perhaps when
patients are dying, they suddenly
acquire a certain celebrity
and become popular!

So much camouflage about patients,
the massive boredom and futility
of dying and of visiting the dying,
so much camouflage about telling

patients the truth, when truth
to tell, those who know that
they are going down the pan
could not care less what you say
– could they? – as long as you
do not abuse them, treat them
cruelly or as if they do not count
when they are beginning to understand
perfectly well that they no longer count.

So you can say what you damn well
please, even though, invariably and
perhaps inevitably, you insult their
intelligence and your own, much of the time.

This necessarily hypocritical situation is far too absurd
to be taken seriously when all concerned are taking it
very seriously indeed!

But like crying – instead of crying? – none of this
can be helped. It's all part of the muddle-through
end game in which we all play our scripted parts
to the best – or worst - of our ability. Scripted by
habit, nature, our quota of emotional intelligence
and the language of sickness and death that most
of us inherit or easily fall into, as we disguise our
emotions and keep them suitably clenched like a fist
that never strikes unless in the reflection that we
have of it in our relentlessly clenched-up eyes
that camouflage our hearts in this minefield
that we call a hospital ward.

Don't Ask, Don't Care

What is there to contemplate
in all this?

What is there to think
other than a single
life and death thought?

As cancer chews you up
and spits you out, how to
come to terms with it,
with or without hindsight?

How to get it into perspective
through shredded thoughts
and mangled emotions
in this shrinkage
of your mind
and soul?

There must be a lesson in this somewhere.

But where?

The lesson, for me, is this:
get on and live or die
and don't complain.

Life's a mysterious farce
and you are no exception.

So don't be a bore.
You've never complained before.

Enter into the party spirit.
and play the game!

Don't ask why
that big man in the sky
wants to punish and torture you
before you are through?

Nobody knows the answer
to such questions.

So it's pointless to ask
or to care.

Without Self-Pity

To suffer without any self-pity
is what it takes to beat the boredom
and misery of suffering from ill-health
and to make it sparkle with dignity,
whilst showing defiant indifference
to false hope and despair,
two fellow travellers to be
taken cheerfully with a large
pinch of salt!

It's worth remembering
that the party's not over
until it's finally over,
and that there is always personal
growth to be painfully acquired through
a total absence of remorse or sorrow
in the hearts and minds of all patients
everywhere on the ward and in the world at large
(with whom this message may strike a chord,
however much they must tolerate the intolerable).

Without labouring the point,
there's no harm in letting –
if you can - humour and the spirit
of captain courageous come
to your aid with a compassionate
lack of self-pity that is kind
and gracious to your nearest
and dearest, and good for your
soul and maybe even your
recovery before you are through.

Never forget who you are and were

before your impertinent disease came
along to con you into thinking that
suddenly you are somebody else
entirely, because it's simply not true.
You are who you always have been
regardless of how cancer or anything
else hideously re-arranges you
in its own image that is not
your self-image. It is an image
that has been wrongfully imposed
upon you that you do not have to
accept, as you stick your tongue out
at it, as and when appropriate!

Re-arranged you may be,
but never seriously altered,
fragile you may be, but hard
as spiritual granite also.

There is much more to you
than flesh and blood and,
as we know, we must all take
our chances in this life
and not count the cost.

Question-Mark Days

In my question-mark days,
when I consulted my tongue
all I could feel was intolerable
soreness until, later on, all I could
taste was unrelenting bitterness
for several months in the black
swamp of my mouth.

Gob smacked by bitter remarks
that rejected my taste buds, I also
lost my voice and questioned whether
it would come back again, just as
I questioned if I would learn to
swallow again, just as everyone
questioned whether
I would live or die.

The first time that I returned to eating solids
it took me an hour and a half to swallow half
a mug of soup, as I gritted my teeth and my heart
through the pain that questioned my tenacity (as did I).
Waiting for me to finish eating - in the paint-stripper
of my mouth - was like watching paint dry!

As for drinking delicious wines,
that was like savouring poison!

There were so many acutely dispiriting
questions in those deeply disillusioning
and depressing question-mark days
during the first two years of my recovery,
after the cancer specialists had scoured
my mouth and throat with their steel wool,

strangled my voice to death,
straightened out my tongue
and ironed it neat and tidy,
together with my crumpled
mouth that had been creased
this way and that….. with questions
about whether I would ever eat,
drink or speak again.

But now, more than four years later,
I am savouring the finest wines,
eating spicy and flavoursome meals,
speaking out loud all over again,
and reading a cancer poem
to members of parliament
and the medical profession
in the House of Commons
at the 2007 launch of Britain's
Mouth Cancer Awareness Week.

The question-mark days do seem to be –
fingers crossed - receding into the past.

Cancer Awareness Weeks

To those who ask - what is the point of cancer awareness? -
the answer is that it helps uninformed people come to realise
what is happening when and where it is happening
so that they can clearly see

that Big Bad cancer is making a horrible mess
of too many people's lives. This comes as a nasty surprise
to those who do not fully comprehend how sickening
and devastating cancer can be.

The point of making the unaware aware
is to get them to stop and think and perhaps spare
some time to help devise a plan, before it is too late,
to beat this disease from hell instead of leaving it to fate.

This is the whole point of an awareness week,
when cancer experts and others turn out to speak
in order to get their message over to a public
that is increasingly becoming fatally sick
with this dreadful illness called cancer
that is putting 1 in 3 of us in danger.

Unless those with the knowledge share what they know,
then the public won't understand which way to go.
It will not be particularly concerned
about what it has never learned.

So let the cancer awareness weeks beat the drum
before, by cancer, we are all undone.
Let the public not be kept in the dark
about cancer not being a stroll through the park!

Let poetry, medicine and prose unite

as, together, they fight the good fight!

Complexity Theory

Be warned! This is a poem
about complexity theory,
so be prepared for
a long haul
on the subject
of molecules.

According to this theory,
the question is not why
do things go wrong
with our health,
but why
do they
not?

As you might expect,
this is one hell
of a theory!

Why does it take only one molecule
going absent without leave,
or wrong, to cause
big bad cancer?

Don't ask the medical scientists
because they do not know,
bless them. But they are
the only ones trying
to find out and before
long they may very well
know the answer.

They know that it does take

only one molecule, but they
do not know why.

Nobody knows why.

Considering that we have trillions of molecules
in each of our bodies -more than ten thousand
billion! – it is perhaps hardly surprising that
so many of them and the multiplying cells
to which they give rise do go wrong,
at least 2,000 of which
turn to cancer when
they overproduce
and run wild.

The human body is not
such a perfect construct
as we would wish.

On the contrary,
it is a perverse
construct.

The concept of trillions of molecules
in a single human being is mind-boggling
and one might ask, not how come there is
so much cancer about, but how come there
is so little, in view of the awesome enormity
and complexity of the human cell structure?

Why should we not get cancer?

A body cell is a life-giving microscopic unit

of living matter, at the centre of which there is
a positively charged nucleus, and around which
other cells are spawned. But the problem is that
not all of these other cells are spawned normally.
Some come out abnormally and it is the abnormal
cells – the monster Jekyll and Hyde cells – that kill
off the normal cells, putting cancer patients on the rack
as they do so. Our insides are swamped in a sea
of molecules that float around like frogspawn,
providing the outer walls and interiors
of our body cells, furnishing them with
a nucleus and also with genes that characterise
these cells in so many different ways.

Our genes are supposed to come in pairs
and they are housed in their nucleus –
each human being has 23 pairs of genes –
but our cells have dual personalities,
some of which are gross and monstrous,
just as we all have dual personalities
that are capable of good and bad
or contradictory things in this life,
as if to suggest that we are in fact
programmed to be contradictory.

It is when our good cells go to the bad
and turn themselves into one or more
of the 200 or 2,000 murderous cancers
of which they are capable on the darker
side of our biology that we are in trouble!

These bad cells don't come in pairs, as intended,
but in hideous bundles, like fungi growing
on other plants or decaying matter,

like toad stalls.

When you get oral cancer it is like having
a monstrous toad stall choking your mouth
and throat!

The fact is that there are all sorts of monster
cells lurking deep down inside us
that can pounce at any time.

It's as if we are designed from birth to be
our own worst enemies – at our own throats
if we don't watch out – and some of us more
so than others and through no fault of our own.

Ominously there is a sleeping enemy within
where there are more things to go wrong
on account of having so many cells – think
of modern automobiles, for example, with
all their clever electronics, or computers –
so it really is a wonder, maybe, that more
things do not go wrong.

Some people believe that things go wrong because
we eat the wrong foods, but one hears that only a
quarter of cancers in the UK are related to
diets. No doubt the secret to the alarming
puzzle has to be in our DNA, an answer
that is perhaps 10 or 20 years away.

There is programmed into us, Matthew Arnold's
eternal note of sadness that Sophocles heard
long ago on the Aegean, complete with the
clash of those 'ignorant armies' within

the cell structure of our bodies,
and when you get cancer you are
on a steep learning curve that is deeply
interesting and thought provoking,
full of ugly fascination!

And here ends my story,
a poetic case study
of an oral cancer patient,
sprinkled with poetic
concepts in amongst
the scientific detail,
to demonstrate that
poetry can indeed
comprehend science
whilst also
informing it.

Laughter the Best Medicine

We are buggered
one way or another
whatever we do,
whatever we eat,
however we live.

If our insides don't get us,
then the polluted outer environment
and global warming, or our enemies,
certainly will when things go wrong
for us, when fate may get us also,
just like our cells and our genes
will get us, but not without having
a good laugh at our expense.

Listen: life is a seriously absurd joke
sick or otherwise - so enjoy it –
and laughter is the best medicine,
however black or blue,
satirical or otherwise

So it makes sense to see
the funny side of cancer
and ourselves!

Beats crying any day.

Morbid Anatomies

Gift-wrapped anatomies
that are tied with pretty ribbons
and come with chocolate box
pictures of smiling health
are seldom full of goodies!

On the contrary, they are full
of future decay and disease
and so many nasty surprises,
as quietly approaching death
and decline from the far distance
of our morbid bodily structures
make their invisible mark
virtually without notice until
we notice what we notice!

These anatomies are full
of pre-destined gloom
and doom that contradicts
the notion that all is well
with us and the world!

Clearly they are having us on,
but to what schizophrenic purpose?

A Fake Remedy?

Of all the medications and treatments
that can relieve our suffering and pain
there is but one that can do so
like no other.

But it goes against our sentiments,
our natural inclinations, and all our moral grain
in the tiresome medical game that we play in the slow
agony of fatal sickness and disease, until the party's over.

Yet there is a cure for all that and, unless it's quackery,
why must we prolong our misery,
as we lose our dignity and wait and see?

Of course the word nostrum cannot be ruled out,
as we gasp our last breath, and shout our last shout.

Cancer at Both Ends

Prostate keyhole surgery is not exactly a doddle.
Naked and frozen between your legs, you wobble
and shake like a jelly, as nurses quickly smother you
with blankets to keep you warm and you turn blue
with cold, while the surgeon quietly freezes your
balls off, leaving you to wonder what more
trouble there is in store!

Maybe I felt the cold more than others because I had
already had a major 8-hour operation for a Big Bad
cancer of the neck, days previously, and had not yet
recovered, but this was an awesome cold not to forget!

You are sedated, but fully conscious as you master your fear,
while the surgeon goes in for the kill with his miniature spear
that glides like an arrow through the keyhole at that tender
tip-top of your cock, to the shock of which you soon surrender,
as his surgical knife travels through to your enlarged and
distorted gland
and sharply removes several fleshy tissues with a skilful deft of
hand,
reducing the size of that formerly pristine walnut that is sitting
beneath your king-size sac - between the twin sewers that it's
invading -
putting pressure on your urinary tact, squashing and preventing
urine from flowing freely from your beleaguered bladder,
which is why you have found it impossible - or harder -
to have a pee when you needed to pass water.

Your prostate gland – that secretes the magical alkaline fluids
into your

excited semen during the thrill and spill of ejaculation, to cries of 'more,

more, more' from your loved one - can turn very nasty and ugly indeed,

and counter with 'less, less!' It can strangle your urethra tube, the need

of which in your penis is beyond dispute! So here is a gland, the correction

of which is essential for you to pass water and enjoy your precious erection,

after the medics have bored a hole through it and cut its saggy old bag

down to size, because it has become overblown and is suddenly a drag

on your urethra, as result of too much wear and tear, becoming a gross

enlargement that is threatening your health and coming very close

to robbing you of your sexual contentment – your nicety – no less.

So you'd better have the operation, I guess!

As we see, there are occasions when shape and form are everything.

More art and less substance are required for a man's ding-a-ling!

It's as if this gland beneath your bladder is taking the piss,
as your bag-like sac begins to boo and hiss.

It is as if your body parts have a cruel sense of humour and satire

all their own, laughing their heads off as you sink into the
mire!

It's not easy for patients to imagine or to understand
what is happening to them when the all-powerful hand
of the surgeon-god is upon them, not easy for them
to comprehend how he can see what he can see when
miniscule pin-head cameras have also been inserted inside
them through the keyhole, with which to guide
the spear and the surgeon's hand
and keep it on target as planned.

Only by paying keen and determined attention
can sedated patients achieve comprehension!

I had a litre and a half of urine that could not be released
from my bladder, as well as some quite possibly diseased
tissues that could have turned cancerous, which was another
reason for scraping these tissues away in order not to discover
a far more lethal problem long after the surgery was over.

Watching shavings of tissue being taken from your prick
certainly makes you queasy if not positively sick!

The surgeon puts them carefully into a tray
that you can see for yourself before it's taken away.

It is a delicate task, gliding through that inner tube
of your prick with a painfully sharp and rude
little instrument that is going to cut your prostate
down to size and leave you in a bloody state
for days afterwards, as you piss your pink champagne
and with much soreness and a certain amount of pain.

Prostate surgery can easily lead to pissy incontinence

or, in the event of collateral damage, sexual impotence,
which is why one needs a skilled and experienced urologist
master-craftsman at the very top of the professional list,
not one of the lesser, ham-fisted kind,
who leaves a trail of destruction behind!

So talk around and shop around, find out who's who,
before you finally decide who will do for you.

Some are at the very top of their exalted profession
and considerably better than others without question,
but not all have perfectly safe or particularly gifted hands,
so they may have made a mess of several prostate glands!

As you see, there is a lot more to keyhole prostate surgery
than neatly inserting a little key in the lock! There is misery
and mystery, discovery and astonishing medical mastery,
all of which is a lot better than full-scale prostatectomy
that can result in butchery!

Full-scale prostatectomy – wounding surgery with its large
open
cuts for a complete removal of the prostate gland, which is
when
you loose so much more blood and experience a full ration of
pain –
may leave you with private parts that will never be the same
again
and it can keep you in hospital for much longer, perhaps 7-10
days
before convalescing for some 6-12 weeks. In so many hideous
ways
this is seriously painful. But keyhole incisions avoid the
painful

cuts of the prostatectomy and, because the key-surgery is minimal,
you can be out of hospital the same or the next day, although
you will take to your bed for 2/3 days maybe, and when you go
to the loo you may pass bloody urine perhaps for about a week.
Keyhole prostate surgery is the very latest method that will seek
to minimise the pain and maximise the gain, but it is
a sophisticated form of torture for all that, it really is!
It may be called 'gold standard,'
but it will hit you hard!

I put off having my prostate surgery for fear of finishing up
incontinent or impotent in the event of having been sold a pup
by an incompetent surgeon, but the keyhole that I eventually had
left me in pretty good shape and not feeling too bad.

I was in and out of hospital the same day, which is just as well,
because I had only just completed the aforesaid operation from hell
on my neck to remove a cancerous lump, and I then went into six
weeks of radiotherapy to my mouth and throat! Such an untimely mix
of treatments and operations – cancer at both ends, if you don't watch out –
from one operation and treatment to the next. Nothing to crow about!

But, neither incontinent nor impotent in my 68th year, I can now piss

like a bull at a gate! Thankfully there's nothing any longer hit
or miss
when I pass urine, but semen no longer erupts forcefully like
magma
when getting one's leg over. It implodes instead of coming
insider her!
One can only come internally, within one's own tool,
which is far less messy, but just as pleasurable, as a rule!

Having survived cancer of the mouth for four years now,
and prostate keyhole surgery likewise, I understand how
one can endure the unendurable
and (hopefully!) cure the incurable.

I also realise how much worse it could have been to have gone
almost down
the pan with two different cancers at both ends, when that
grotesque clown
called fate gave me looks that kill, only to find that the feeling
was mutual,
as my surgeons, doctors, carer-wife and I made known our
refusal.

Cancer at one end was certainly bad enough,
but at both ends would have been rough
justice and a double whammy
that was very far from funny.

A Finger up the Bum

A lubricated finger up the bum
sounds like a needless indignity
or perhaps an illicit sexual pleasure
for those who are that way inclined.

But it is otherwise
a routine necessity
if you happen to have
an enlarged prostate
that needs to be felt
in order to be confirmed.

However, this solitary finger
of suspicion is only
the beginning.

There's more yet
from this fickle finger
of pleasure or is it fate?

What follows is a little piercing arrow
that goes up the bum likewise,
with a miniscule insect camera-head
delicately inserted in its protective helmet
like a miniaturised miner's Davie-lamp
to show the way in the dark and to televise
your prostate on a TV screen, so that you
can watch the progress of the arrow as it
travels inside you, as you lie naked
and face down on the surgeon's couch
for ease of access to your back passage.

This insect camera-probe is everything.
It is a light carrying a filament
and a pipette for extracting
the fleshy tissues required
for the purposes of biopsy,
with the knife (or arrow)
is in the tip of the probe.

The probe's arrow shoots out from
what looks like the barrel of a tiny
revolver in the surgeon's hand that
triggers it, as it penetrates your back
passage in order to locate your prostate
gland, from which it takes slithers
and shavings of tissue to put them under
the microscope and see whether or not
they are cancerous.

My tissues were not exactly cancerous.
They were described as 'benign,'
as opposed to unfriendly
and positively cancerous
therefore!

Like sleeping dogs
they were friendly enough
unless and until they were woken!

So the suspicious patch
on my enlarged prostate
was referred to as a 'freckle,'
rather than a cancer, but it needed
to be kept under regular observation
for fear of its ceasing to be a freckle

and turning itself into a cancer instead.

For this reason, regular blood tests
were required, so that blood could be
fractionated from my sperm in that
particularly bloody and spermy
part of the body in which
a prostate cancer can travel
swiftly and spread through
the blood stream
like wildfire, should it
suddenly strike.

As it happened, my cancer struck elsewhere
and without warning or any prior symptoms -
in my mouth at the opposite end of my body! -
as if to suggest that it was a mischievous body
that was playing games with me and my doctors,
tricking us into thinking one thing and sending
us off in the wrong direction entirely!

Again, it was as if my body was mocking me
and having a good laugh at my expense……

But my surgeon was so proud of his pesky little finger,
as he waved it in the air, gleefully explaining how many
bums it had penetrated over the years. But not without
adding a note of caution! Which was that even though
his finger's track record was good, there was no guarantee
that it would accurately feel and confirm an enlarged prostate
every single time. His finger was not infallible!
It could occasionally get a prostate wrong.

But where would we be without it?

He seemed to think that feeling an enlarged prostate with
a finger was an art – no doubt it is – a case of *ledgerdemain*.

To get him off the subject,
I tried to interest him
in my penis, telling him that
it had also penetrated a great many
intimate bodily places over the years,
thrusting and rotating around inside them,
just like his finger, and that it too was not
infallible. It did sometimes get a few things
wrong, but no often!

But he was not in the least interested in that.

Lucky Sod

What a lucky sod I am,
Oh what a lucky sod I am,
I could have had a face to stop a clock
I could have had a prostate op' to wreck my cock
I could have had absolutely nothing of which to complain
I could have been in deep denial about the anger and the pain
I could have been silenced by being misaccused of self-pity
I could have been feeling good instead of shitty
I could have had a disease to make me croak
I could have been a really lucky bloke
Without any teeth to give me hell
Or cancer to make me unwell.
Sans teeth
Sans everything
Oh what a lucky sod I am!
Oh, oh, oh what a lovely war…
I think we've all been here before!

Between His Legs

Between his legs, a skull and cross-bones
beg the question, as the sharp teeth of cancer
bite into his balls and he sees his face staring
at him in horror out of the shrinking manhood
of his testicles, no longer the fatal fascination
of the opposite sex, no longer the sexual power
of his physical being that is shrinking fast
with his life and his no longer proud
or pleasurably erect penis.

Between his legs, prostate and testicular cancer
seem to have him by the balls, as these diseases
take the piss with their incontinence and impotence,
their slugs and snails and puppy dog's tails.

There is such an irony and a mockery
and final insult to that former manhood
between his legs where a ghastly skull
and cross-bones haunt him and his carers
with that emblem of death and of piracy.

There is simply too much to disgust
and to terrify him between his legs,
as he keeps his calm and his cool
and lets a wry smile pass his lips,
as he realises only too well that,
truth to tell, the joke's on him!

Poetry and Cancer

What is poetry and free verse
if not painting framed pictures with words?
What is cancer if not an ugly picture
to which we had all better pay attention
in fact and/or fiction?

Thought Waves

It is the bitter-sweet nature of language
that makes poetry, as well as a difference
in format on the printed page in favour
of a poem lining up the emotions in rows
and blocks of patterned thoughts that flow
from line to line and left to right and back again,
image by image and insight by insight, in a more
cogent and precise way than prose allows, so that
ideas and feelings can be encapsulated and swiftly
delivered much more clearly and maybe dramatically,
both literally and verbally, in precious thought waves,
sometimes powerful and other times subtle or magical,
as they reveal a mental map that we call poetry.

The Acid Test of Cancer Poetry

Because words can seriously affect
your heart and destroy your immunity
to human emotions, as Elma Mitchell
always said, then nakedly revealing
poems can be dangerous, not least
cancer poems that tell truths that
are as fatal as the disease itself,
as they hold up a reflective mirror
to ugly cancer, a mirror that is just
as painful as the disease itself,
with its awareness of a compelling
need for moral victories in the face
of too many physical defeats.

Such poetry is the acid test
of mind over matter that says
never mind and no matter!

Dedication

To cancer sufferers everywhere and to the staff of the maxillofacial department at University College Hospital in London, in particular to
surgeons Lawrence Newman and Nicholas Kalavrezos, Dr Prior and Professor Michele Saunders who, for their sins, seem to have saved
my life. To my wife also, who nursed and cared for me good and proper for two long years.

Other Books of Poetry by Bob Crew Currently in the Bookstalls and on Amazon

Sea Poems, co-published by Sheridan House in New York and Seafarer Books in the UK.

Surviving Schizophrenia and Mind & Soul Poetry, published by Chipmunka Publishing in London.

Lightning Source UK Ltd.
Milton Keynes UK
UKHW051107060223
416527UK00011B/490